DASH DIET

COOKBOOK FOR BEGINNERS

RECIPES IN THIS COOKBOOK WRITE JUST FOR TWO, SIMPLE AND EASY TO FOLLOW. DISCOVER THE BEST WEIGHT LOSS SOLUTION ON THE MARKET, FIND TRICKS AND TIPS TO LOWER YOUR BLOOD PRESSURE. DO NOT WAIT! ACT NOW, START YOUR DASH DIET !

TABLE OF CONTENTS

CHAPTER 1

INTRODUCTION

If you're ready to get started, the Dash Diet Cookbook is here to help. There's something for everyone in this book, from breakfast items to dinner side dishes. Feel great about what you eat with the Dash Diet Cookbook!

This guide is your guide to the Dash Diet Cookbook. If you have been following the diet for any amount of time, you will appreciate the information in this guide. Take advantage of the resources provided in this guide to ensure that you succeed on a diet.

The diet focuses on certain food groups for specific reasons: Fruits and vegetables give you the magnesium and potassium your body needs, and low-fat dairy products provide calcium. However, every food you eat should have a purpose, and that's the essential principle of the DASH diet: eat well, so you feel well.

A DASH diet can be easily integrated into daily life simply because it uses foods that are available in conventional grocery stores. Then, depending on your calorie requirement, the amounts consumed of the individual foods result.

WHAT CAN I EAT?

Allowed foods are:
> plenty of fresh vegetables, especially lots of greens - almost without restriction
> Fresh fruit
> lean meats, especially white meat (chicken, turkey)
> Whole grain / whole grain products
> fish
> Protein-rich foods
> Foods with unsaturated and healthy fats such as nuts and avocados
> Healthy oils with an optimal Omega3 / 6 ratio such as olive oil and coconut oil
> Lean dairy products
> Nuts, seeds, legumes

In small amounts:
> alcohol
> coffee
> animal fats, especially red meat
> Sweets and sugar

Avoid as much as possible:
> Ready meals and canned food
> Sausages
> Bakery products
> hydrogenated vegetable fats such as palm fat
> Sunflower oil (poor omega3 / 6 ratio)
> pickled and smoked foods

How DASH Diet Help You Lose Weight And Lower Blood Pressure

Despite not being specifically designed for weight loss, the Dash Diet does indeed help to trim down your weight through various indirect means.

While the DASH diet does not include stress reductions in calories, it influences you to fill up your diet with very nutrient-dense food instead of calorie-rich food, which quickly helps to shed a few pounds!

Since you will be on a heavy diet of veggies and fruits, you will be consuming lots of fiber, which is also believed to help weight loss.

Aside from that, the diet also helps to control your appetite since cleaner, and nutrient-dense foods will keep you satisfied throughout the day! In addition, lower food intake will further contribute to weight loss.

And while you are at it, the program will indirectly encourage you to carry out a daily workout to keep your body healthy and fit. Therefore, following the DASH Diet program while working out will significantly enhance the effectiveness of the program.

Understanding the food groups

To keep things simple, let me break down the food groups to understand the food regime of the program better.

Eat as much as you want

Grains, such as barley, wheat bread, wheat pasta, etc.

Meats, such as eggs, lean beef, lean chicken, lean pork

Seafood, such as fish, Shrimp, and Salmon

Fruits such as apples, bananas, cherries, grapes, blackberries, mangoes, etc.

Vegetables such as artichokes, broccoli, Brussels sprouts, carrots, bell peppers, green beans, etc.

Limit Your Servings

Healthy vegetable oils, such as canola, corn, olive, etc.

Condiments

Dairy such as Greek yogurt, skim milk, low-fat milk, low-fat cheese

Nuts, legumes, and seeds such as almonds, cashews, flax seeds, hazelnuts, lentils, pecans, kidney beans

Red meats

Eat Rarely

Sweets such as beverages, jams, jellies, sugars, sweet yogurt

Saturated fats such as bacon, cholesterol, coconuts, fatty meats

Sodium-rich foods such as canned fruits, canned vegetables, gravy pizza, etc.

Understanding daily proportions

Controlling your daily portions is crucial when it comes to the Dash Diet program. While the critical component here is to keep your sodium intake at a low level, there are other things that you must consider.

So, to properly maintain your DASH diet, you should:

Consume more fruits, low-fat dairy foods, and vegetables

Eat more whole-grain foods, nuts, poultry, and fish

Try to limit sodium, sugary drinks, sweets, and red meat, such as beef/pork, etc.

Research has shown that you will get results within just two weeks!

Alternatively, a different form of diet known as DASH-Sodium calls for cutting down sodium to about 1,500 mg per day (which weighs about 2/3 teaspoon per day)

Generally speaking, the suggested DASH routine includes:

Daily 7-8 servings of grains

Daily 4-5 servings of vegetables

Daily 4-5 servings of fruits

Daily 2-3 servings of low-fat/ fat-free dairy products

Daily 2 or fewer servings of meat/fish/poultry

4-5 servings per week of nuts, dry beans, and seeds

Daily 2-3 servings of fats and oil

And just to give you an idea of what "Each" serving means, here are a few pointers.

The following quantities are to be considered as one serving:

½ cup of cooked rice/pasta

1 slice of bread

1 cup of raw fruit or veggies

½ cup of cooked fruit or veggies

8 ounces of milk

3 ounces of cooked meat

1 teaspoon of olive oil/ or any healthy oil

3 ounces of tofu

1 slice of bread
1 cup of raw fruit or veggies
½ cup of cooked fruit or veggies
8 ounces of milk
3 ounces of cooked meat
1 teaspoon of olive oil/ or any healthy oil
3 ounces of tofu

Some salt alternatives to know about

Letting go of salt might be a little bit difficult for people going into this diet for the first time.
To make the process a little bit easier, here are some great salt alternatives that you should know about!
Some of them are used in the recipes in our book, and you may use them if needed.

Sunflower Seeds
Sunflower seeds are fantastic salt alternatives, and they give a nice nutty and slightly sweet flavor. You may use the seeds raw or roasted.
Fresh Squeezed Lemon
Lemon is believed to be a nice hybrid between citron and bitter orange. These are packed with Vitamin C, which helps to neutralize damaging free radicals from the system.

Onion Powder
Onion powder is a dry and ground spice made out of an onion bulb for those you don't know. The powder is mainly used for seasoning in many herbs! Keep in mind that onion powder and onion salt are two different things.
We are using onion powder here. They sport a nice mix of sweet, spicy, and a bit of an earthy flavor.

Black Pepper Powder
Black pepper powder is also a salt alternative that is native to India. You may use them by grinding whole peppercorns!

Cinnamon
Cinnamon is a very well-known and savory spice that comes from the inner bark of trees. Two varieties of cinnamon include Ceylon and Chinese, and they sport a sharp, warm and sweet flavor.

Flavored Vinegar
As we call it in our book, fruit-infused vinegar or a flavored vinegar is a mixture of vinegar combined with fruits to give a nice flavor. These are excellent ingredients to add a bit of flavor to meals without salt. Experiment to find the perfect fruit blend for you.
As for the process of making the vinegar:
- Wash your fruits and slice them well
- Place ½ cup of your fruit in a mason jar
- Top them up with white wine vinegar (or balsamic vinegar)
- Allow them to sit for two weeks or so
- Strain and use as needed

The Health Benefits of Dash Diet
Before you move forward, let me share some of the excellent health benefits you will enjoy while you are on the program.

Lower Blood Pressure

This is perhaps the main reason why the DASH diet was even invented!

Salt is believed to be very closely related to increasing blood pressure. Therefore, the purpose of the DASH diet is to closely monitor the intake of salt and reduce it to very minute levels and improve your overall blood pressure.

Aside from the salt itself, the DASH diet also helps control potassium, magnesium, and calcium, which altogether plays a significant role in lowering blood pressure!

A balanced diet also helps control cholesterol and fat levels in your system, preventing atherosclerosis, which further helps keep the arteries healthy and strain-free.

Helps Control Diabetes

Since the Dash Diet helps to eliminate empty carbohydrates and starchy food from your diet while avoiding simple sugars, a delicate balance between the glucose and insulin level of the body is created that helps prevent diabetes.

Also:

- Lowers blood pressure
- Helps to lower cholesterol levels
- Helps in weight loss
- Gives you a healthier heart
- Helps to prevent Osteoporosis
- Helps to improve kidney health
- Helps to prevent cancer
- Helps to control diabetes
- Helps to prevent depression

CHAPTER 2.

BREAKFASTS

TOASTIES

Preparation Time: 30 minutes
Cooking Time: 15-20 minutes
Servings: 2

INGREDIENTS

- ¼ cup of milk or cream
- 2 sausages, boiled
- 3 eggs
- 1 slice of bread, sliced lengthwise
- 4 tablespoons of cheese, grated
- Sea salt to taste
- Chopped fresh herbs and steamed broccoli [optional]

DIRECTIONS

1. Preheat your Air Fryer at 360 °F and set the timer for 5 minutes.
2. In the meantime, scramble the eggs in a bowl and add in the milk.
3. Grease three muffin cups with a cooking spray. Divide the egg mixture into three and pour equal amounts into each cup.
4. Slice the sausages and drop them, along with the slices of bread, into the egg mixture. Add the cheese on top and a little salt as desired.
5. Transfer the cups to the fryer and cook for 15-20 minutes, depending on how firm you would like them. When ready, remove them from the fryer, serve with fresh herbs and steam broccoli if you prefer.
6.

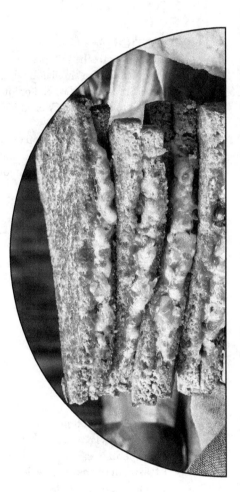

EGG BAKED OMELET

Preparation Time: 15 minutes
Cooking Time: 10 minutes
Servings: 2

INGREDIENTS

- 1 tablespoon of ricotta cheese
- 1 tablespoon of chopped parsley
- 1 tsp. olive oil
- 3 eggs
- ¼ cup chopped spinach
- ¼ cup ricotta cheese
- Salt and pepper to taste

DIRECTIONS

1. Set your Air Fryer at 330 °F and allow it to warm with the olive oil inside.
2. In a bowl, beat the eggs with a fork and sprinkle some salt and pepper as desired.
3. Add in the ricotta, spinach, and parsley and then transfer to the Air Fryer. Cook for 10 minutes before serving.

BREAKFAST OMELET

Preparation Time: 30 minutes
Cooking Time: 15 minutes
Servings: 2

INGREDIENTS

- 1 large onion, chopped
- 2 tablespoons of cheddar cheese, grated
- 3 eggs
- ½ teaspoon of soy sauce
- Salt
- Pepper powder
- Cooking spray

DIRECTIONS

1. In a bowl, mix the salt, pepper powder, soy sauce and eggs with a whisk.
2. Take a small pan small enough to fit inside the Air Fryer and spritz with cooking spray. Spread the chopped onion across the bottom of the pan, and then transfer the pan to the Fryer. Cook at 355°F for 6-7 minutes, ensuring the onions turn translucent.
3. Add the egg mixture on top of the onions, coating everything well. Add the cheese on top, and then resume cooking for another 5 or 6 minutes.
4. Take care when taking the pan out of the fryer. Enjoy with some toasted bread.

NUTRITION

- Calories: 346
- Fat: 11.5 g
- Fiber: 3.4 g
- Carbs: 11.5 g
- Protein: 5.6 g

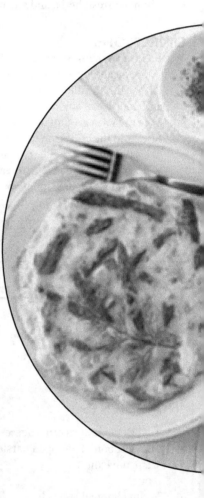

COFFEE DONUTS

Preparation Time: 20 minutes
Cooking Time: 10 minutes
Servings: 2

INGREDIENTS

- 1 cup of almond flour
- ¼ cup of stevia
- ½ teaspoon of salt
- 1 teaspoon of baking powder
- 1 tablespoon of aquafaba
- 1 tablespoon of sunflower oil
- ¼ cup of coffee

DIRECTIONS

1. In a large bowl, combine the stevia, salt, flour, and baking powder.
2. Add in the coffee, aquafaba, and sunflower oil and mix until a dough is formed. Leave the dough to rest in and the refrigerator.
3. Set your Air Fryer at 400 °F to heat up.
4. Remove the dough from the fridge and divide up, kneading each section into a doughnut.
5. Put the doughnuts inside the air fryer, ensuring not to overlap any. Fry for 6 minutes. Do not shake the basket to make sure the doughnuts hold their shape.

NUTRITION

- Calories: 346
- Fat: 11.5 g
- Fiber: 3.4 g
- Carbs: 11.5 g
- Protein: 5.6 g

TACO WRAPS

Preparation Time: 30 minutes
Cooking Time: 15 minutes
Servings: 2

INGREDIENTS

- 1 tablespoon of water
- 4 pieces of commercial vegan nuggets, chopped
- 1 small yellow onion, diced
- 1 small red bell pepper, chopped
- 2 cobs of grilled corn kernels
- 4 large corn tortillas
- Mixed greens for garnish

DIRECTIONS

1. Preheat your Air Fryer at 400 °F.
2. Over medium heat, water-sauté the nuggets with the onions, corn kernels and bell peppers in a skillet, then remove from the heat.
3. Fill the tortillas with the nuggets and vegetables and fold them up. Transfer to the inside of the fryer and cook for 15 minutes. Once crispy, serve immediately, garnished with the mixed greens.

NUTRITION

- Calories: 287
- Fat: 11.5 g
- Fiber: 3.4 g
- Carbs: 11.5 g
- Protein: 5.6 g

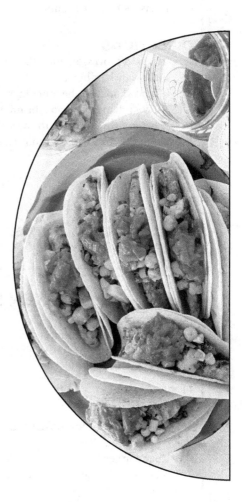

BISTRO WEDGES

Preparation Time: 20 minutes
Cooking Time: 15 minutes
Servings: 2

INGREDIENTS

- 1 lb. of fingerling potatoes, cut into wedges
- 1 teaspoon of extra virgin olive oil
- ½ teaspoon of garlic powder
- Salt and pepper to taste
- ½ cup of raw cashews, soaked in water overnight
- ½ teaspoon of ground turmeric
- ½ teaspoon of paprika
- 1 tablespoon of nutritional yeast
- 1 teaspoon of fresh lemon juice
- 2 tablespoons of to ¼ cup water
- ¼ cup of parmesan cheese

DIRECTIONS

1. Preheat your Air Fryer at 400 °F.
2. In a bowl, toss the potato wedges, olive oil, garlic powder, and salt and pepper, making sure to coat the potatoes well.
3. Transfer the potatoes to the basket of your fryer and fry for 10 minutes.
4. In the meantime, prepare the cheese sauce. Pulse the cashews, turmeric, paprika, nutritional yeast, lemon juice, and water together in a food processor. Add more water to achieve your desired consistency.
5. When the potatoes are finished cooking, move them to a small bowl to fit inside the fryer and add the cheese sauce on top. Cook for an additional 3 minutes.

NUTRITION

- Calories: 346
- Fat: 11.5 g
- Fiber: 3.4 g
- Carbs: 11.5 g
- Protein: 5.6 g

SPINACH BALLS

Preparation Time: 20 minutes
Cooking Time: 10 minutes
Servings: 2

INGREDIENTS

- 1 carrot, peeled and grated
- 1 package fresh spinach, blanched and chopped
- ½ onion, chopped
- 1 egg, beaten
- ½ teaspoon of garlic powder
- 1 teaspoon of garlic, minced
- 1 teaspoon of salt
- ½ teaspoon of black pepper
- 1 tablespoon of nutritional yeast
- 1 tablespoon of almond flour
- 2 slices of bread, toasted

DIRECTIONS

1. In a food processor, pulse the toasted bread to form breadcrumbs. Transfer into a shallow dish or bowl.
2. In a bowl, mix all the other ingredients.
3. Use your hands to shape the mixture into small-sized balls. Roll the balls in the breadcrumbs, ensuring to cover them well.
4. Put in the Air Fryer and cook at 390°F for 10 minutes.

NUTRITION

- Calories: 278
- Fat: 11.5 g
- Fiber: 3.4 g
- Carbs: 11.5 g
- Protein: 5.6 g

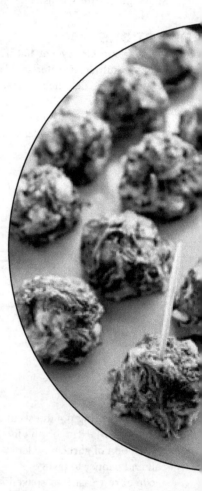

CHEESE & CHICKEN SANDWICH

Preparation Time: 15 minutes
Cooking Time: 5-7 minutes
Servings: 2

INGREDIENTS

- 1/3 cup of chicken, cooked and shredded
- 2 mozzarella slices
- 1 hamburger bun
- ¼ cup of cabbage, shredded
- 1 teaspoon of mayonnaise
- 2 teaspoon of butter
- 1 teaspoon of olive oil
- ½ teaspoon of balsamic vinegar
- 1/4 teaspoon of smoked paprika
- ¼ teaspoon of black pepper
- ¼ teaspoon of garlic powder
- Pinch of salt

DIRECTIONS

1. Preheat your Air Fryer at 370 °F.
2. Apply some butter to the outside of the hamburger bun with a brush.
3. In a bowl, coat the chicken with garlic powder, salt, pepper, and paprika.
4. In a separate bowl, stir together the mayonnaise, olive oil, cabbage, and balsamic vinegar to make coleslaw.
5. Slice the bun in two. Start building the sandwich, starting with the chicken, followed by the mozzarella, the coleslaw, and finally the top bun.
6. Transfer the sandwich to the fryer and cook for 5 – 7 minutes.

NUTRITION

- Calories: 314
- Fat: 11.5 g
- Fiber: 3.4 g
- Carbs: 11.5 g
- Protein: 5.6 g

BACON & HORSERADISH CREAM

Preparation Time: 1 hour 40 minutes
Cooking Time: 1 hour 40 minutes
Servings: 2

INGREDIENTS

- ½ lb. of thick cut bacon, diced
- 2 tablespoon of butter
- 2 shallots, sliced
- ½ cup of milk
- 1 ½ lb. of Brussels sprouts, halved
- 2 tablespoon of almond flour
- 1 cup of heavy cream
- 2 tablespoon of prepared horseradish
- ½ tablespoon of fresh thyme leaves
- 1/8 teaspoon of ground nutmeg
- 1 tablespoon of olive oil
- ½ teaspoon of sea salt
- Ground black pepper to taste
- ½ cup of water

DIRECTIONS

1. Preheat your Air Fryer at 400 °F.
2. Coat the Brussels sprouts with olive oil and sprinkle some salt and pepper on top. Transfer to the fryer and cook for a half-hour. Give them a good stir at the halfway point, then take them out of the fryer and set to the side.
3. Put the bacon in the fryer's basket and pour the water into the drawer underneath to catch the fat. Cook for 10 minutes, stirring 2 or 3 times throughout the cooking time.
4. When 10 minutes are up, add in the shallots. Cook for a further 10 – 15 minutes, making sure the shallots soften up and the bacon turns brown. Add some more pepper and remove. Leave to drain on some paper towels.
5. Melt the butter over the stove or in the microwave before adding in the flour and mixing with a whisk. Slowly add in the heavy cream and milk, and continue to whisk for another 3 – 5 minutes, making sure the mixture thickens.
6. Add the horseradish, thyme, salt, and nutmeg, and stir well once more.
7. Take a 9" x 13" baking dish and grease it with oil. Preheat your oven to 350 °F.
8. Put the Brussels sprouts in the baking dish and spread them across the base. Pour over the cream sauce and then top with a layer of bacon and shallots.
9. Cook in the oven for a half-hour and enjoy.

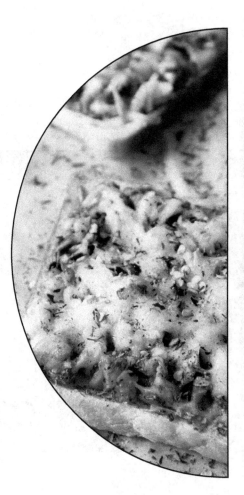

VEGETABLE TOAST

Preparation Time: 25 minutes
Cooking Time: 15 minutes
Servings: 2

INGREDIENTS

- 4 slices of bread
- 1 red bell pepper, cut into strips
- 1 cup of a sliced button or cremini mushrooms
- 1 small yellow squash, sliced
- 2 green onions, sliced
- 1 tablespoon of olive oil
- 2 tablespoons of softened butter
- ½ cup of soft goat cheese

DIRECTIONS

1. Drizzle the Air Fryer with olive oil and preheat to 350 °F.
2. Put the red pepper, green onions, mushrooms, and squash inside the fryer and give them a stir and cook for 7 minutes, shaking the basket once throughout the cooking time. Ensure the vegetables become tender.
3. Remove the vegetables and set them aside.
4. Spread some butter on the slices of bread and transfer to the Air Fryer, butter side-up. Brown for 2 to 4 minutes.
5. Remove the toast from the fryer and top with goat cheese and vegetables. Serve warm.

CHAPTER 3.
SEAFOOD

BAKED COD WITH PARMESAN & ALMONDS

Preparation Time: 40 minutes
Cooking Time: 30 minutes
Servings: 2

INGREDIENTS

- 2 cod fillets
- 1 cup of Brussels sprouts
- 1 tablespoon of butter, melted
- Salt and black pepper to taste
- 1 cup of crème Fraiche
- 2 tablespoons of Parmesan cheese, grated
- 2 tablespoons of shaved almonds

DIRECTIONS

1. Toss the fish fillets and Brussels sprouts in butter and season with salt and black pepper to taste.
2. Spread in a greased baking dish.
3. Mix the crème Fraiche with Parmesan cheese, pour and smear the cream on the fish.
4. Bake in the oven for 25 minutes at 400 °F until golden brown on top, take the dish out, sprinkle with the almonds and bake for another 5 minutes. Best served hot.

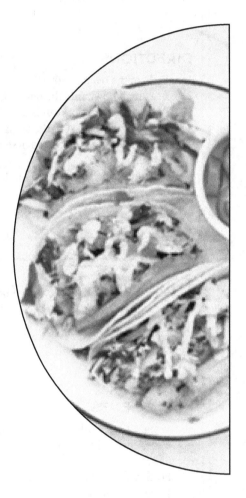

FISH TACOS WITH SLAW, LEMON AND CILANTRO

Preparation Time: 20 minutes
Cooking Time: 15 minutes
Servings: 2

INGREDIENTS

- 1 tablespoon of olive oil
- 1 teaspoon of chili powder
- 2 halibut fillets, skinless, sliced
- 2 low carb tortillas
- Slaw
- 2 tablespoons of red cabbage, shredded
- 1 tablespoon of lemon juice
- Salt to taste
- ½ tablespoon of extra-virgin olive oil
- ½ carrot, shredded
- 1 tablespoon of cilantro, chopped
- ¼ tbsp. paprika

DIRECTIONS

1. Combine the red cabbage with salt in a bowl; massage cabbage to tenderize.
2. Add the remaining slaw ingredient, toss to coat, and set aside.
3. Rub the halibut with olive oil, chili powder, and paprika.
4. Heat a grill pan over medium heat.
5. Add the halibut and cook until lightly charred and cooked through, about 3 minutes per side. Divide between the tortillas.
6. Combine all slaw ingredients in a bowl. Split the slaw among the tortillas.

FRIED OYSTERS IN THE OVEN

Preparation Time: 20 minutes
Cooking Time: 30 minutes
Servings: 2

INGREDIENTS

- 3 tablespoons of olive oil
- 1 teaspoon of garlic salt
- 1 teaspoon of freshly ground black pepper
- 1 teaspoon of red pepper flakes
- 2 cups of finely crushed pork rinds
- 24 shucked oysters

DIRECTIONS

1. Preheat the oven to 400 ºF.
2. In a small bowl, mix the olive oil, garlic salt, black pepper, and red pepper flakes.
3. Put the crushed pork rinds in a separate bowl.
4. Dip each oyster first in the oil mixture to coat and then in the pork rinds, turning to coat. Arrange the coated oysters on a baking sheet in a single layer with room in between.
5. Bake in the preheated oven for 30 minutes, or until the pork rind "breading" is browned and crisp. Serve hot.

NUTRITION
- Calories: 230
- Carbs: 5 g
- Fat: 17g
- Fiber: 0 g
- Protein: 15 g

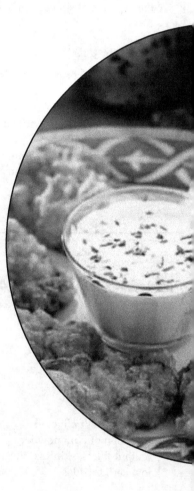

TUNA WITH GREENS AND BLUEBERRIES -ONE POT

Preparation Time: 10 minutes
Cooking Time: 5 minutes
Servings: 2

INGREDIENTS

- ¼ cup of olive oil
- 2 -4-ounces of tuna steaks
- Salt
- Freshly ground black pepper
- Juice of 1 lemon
- 4 cups of salad greens
- ¼ cup of low-carb, dairy-free ranch dressing Tessemae's
- 10 blueberries

DIRECTIONS

1. In a large skillet, heat the olive oil over medium-high heat.
2. Season the tuna steaks generously with salt and pepper, and add them to the skillet. Cook for 2 or 2 ½ minutes on each side to sear the outer edges.
3. Squeeze the lemon over the tuna in the pan and remove the fish
4. To serve, arrange the greens on 2 serving plates. Top each plate with one of the tuna steaks, 2 tablespoons of the ranch dressing, and 10 blueberries.

NUTRITION
- Calories: 549
- Carbs: 7 g
- Fat: 41 g
- Fiber: 3 g
- Protein: 38 g

ROASTED OLD BAY PRAWNS

Preparation Time: 20 minutes
Cooking Time: 15 minutes
Servings: 2

INGREDIENTS

- 3/4 pound of prawns, peeled and deveined
- 1 teaspoon of Old Bay seasoning mix
- 1/2 teaspoon of paprika
- Coarse sea salt and ground black pepper, to taste
- 1 habanero pepper, deveined and minced
- 1 bell pepper, deveined and minced
- 1 cup of pound broccoli florets
- 2 teaspoons of olive oil
- 1 tablespoon of fresh chives, chopped
- 2 slices of lemon for garnish
- 2 dollops of sour cream for garnish

DIRECTIONS

1. Toss the prawns with the Old Bay seasoning mix, paprika, salt, and black pepper. Arrange them on a parchment-lined roasting pan.
2. Add the bell pepper and broccoli.
3. Drizzle the olive oil over everything and transfer the pan to a preheated oven.
4. Roast at 390 ºF for 8 to 11 minutes, turning the pan halfway through the cooking time.
5. Bake until the prawns are pink and cooked through.
6. Serve with fresh chives, lemon, and sour cream.

NUTRITION
- Calories: 269
- Total Fat: 9.6 g
- Carbs: 7.2 g
- Protein: 38.2 g

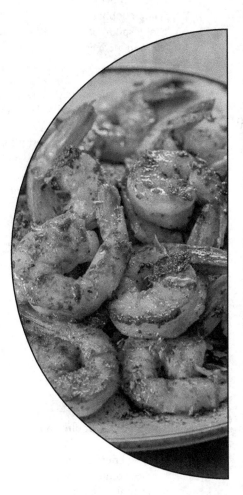

THREE-MINUTE LOBSTER TAIL

Preparation Time: 5 minutes
Cooking Time: 5 minutes
Servings: 2

INGREDIENTS

- 4 cups of bone broth, or water
- 2 lobster tails

DIRECTIONS

1. In a large pot, bring the broth to a boil.
2. While the broth is coming to a boil, use kitchen shears to cut the backside of the lobster shell from end to end.
3. Place the lobster in the boiling broth and bring it back to a boil. Cook the lobster for 3 minutes.
4. Drain and serve immediately.

NUTRITION
- Calories: 154
- Carbs: 0 g
- Fat: 2 g
- Fiber: 0 g
- Protein: 32 g

CRISPY SALMON WITH BROCCOLI & RED BELL PEPPER

Preparation Time: 30 minutes
Cooking Time: 15 minutes
Servings: 2

INGREDIENTS

- 2 salmon fillets
- Salt and black pepper to taste
- 2 tablespoons of mayonnaise
- 2 tablespoons of fennel seeds, crushed
- ½ head of broccoli, cut in florets
- 1 red bell pepper, sliced
- ¼ cup chopped carrots
- 1 tablespoon of olive oil
- 2 lemon wedges

DIRECTIONS

1. Brush the salmon with mayonnaise and season with salt and black pepper.
2. Coat with fennel seeds, place in a lined baking dish and bake for 15 minutes at 370 F.
3. Steam the broccoli and carrot for 3-4 minutes, or until tender, in a pot over medium heat. Heat the olive oil in a saucepan and sauté the red bell pepper for 5 minutes.
4. Stir in the broccoli and turn off the heat. Let the pan sit on the warm burner for 2-3 minutes.
5. Serve with baked salmon garnished with lemon wedges.

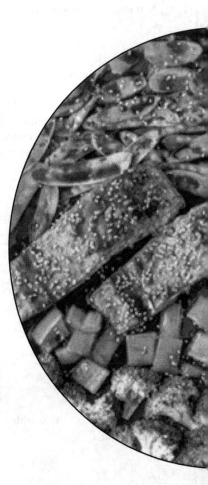

EASY BAKED HALIBUT STEAKS

Preparation Time: 20 minutes
Cooking Time: 15 minutes
Servings: 2

INGREDIENTS

- 2 tablespoons of olive oil
- 2 halibut steaks
- 1 red bell pepper, sliced
- 1 yellow onion, sliced
- 1 teaspoon of garlic, smashed
- 1/2 teaspoon of hot paprika
- Sea salt cracked black pepper, to your liking
- 1 dried thyme sprig, leaves crushed

DIRECTIONS

1. Start by preheating your oven to 390 °F.
2. Then, drizzle the olive oil over the halibut steaks.
3. Place the halibut in a baking dish that is previously greased with a nonstick spray.
4. Top with bell pepper, onion, and garlic.
5. Sprinkle with hot paprika, salt, black pepper, and dried thyme over everything.
6. Bake in the preheated oven for 13 to 15 minutes and serve immediately. Enjoy!

MEDITERRANEAN TILAPIA BAKE

Preparation Time: 20 minutes
Cooking Time: 15 minutes
Servings: 2

INGREDIENTS

- 2 tablespoons of olive oil
- 4 cups of noodles, spiraled zucchini
- ½ pound of whole fresh sardines, gutted and cleaned
- ½ cup of sun-dried tomatoes, drained and chopped
- 1 tablespoon of dill
- 1 garlic clove, minced
- Salt and Black Pepper, to taste

DIRECTIONS

1. Preheat the oven to 350 ºF and line a baking sheet with parchment paper.
2. Arrange the sardines on the dish, drizzle with olive oil, sprinkle with salt and black pepper. Bake in the oven for 10 minutes until the skin is crispy.
3. Warm the oil in a skillet over medium heat and stir-fry the zucchini, garlic, and tomatoes for 5 minutes.
4. Adjust the seasoning.
5. Transfer the sardines to a plate and serve with the veggie pasta.

NUTRITION

- Calories: 232
- Total Fat: 6.7 g
- Carbs: 3.6 g
- Protein: 38.1 g

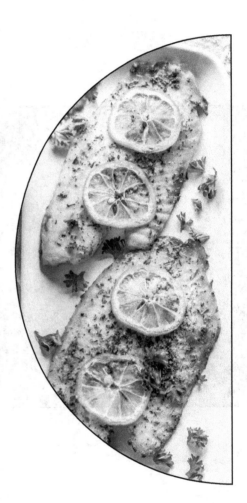

SAUCY COD WITH MUSTARD GREENS

Preparation Time: 20 minutes
Cooking Time: 15 minutes
Servings: 2

INGREDIENTS

- 1 tablespoon of olive oil
- 1 bell pepper, seeded and sliced
- 1 jalapeno pepper, seeded and sliced
- 2 stalks of green onions, sliced
- 1 stalk of green garlic, sliced
- 1/2 cup of fish broth
- 2 cod fish fillets
- 1/2 teaspoon of paprika
- Sea salt and ground black pepper, to season
- 1 cup of mustard greens, torn into bite-sized pieces

DIRECTIONS

1. Heat the olive oil in a Dutch pot over a moderate flame.
2. Now, sauté the peppers, green onions, and garlic until just tender and aromatic.
3. Add in the broth, fish fillets, paprika, salt, black pepper, and mustard greens.
4. Reduce the temperature to medium-low, cover, and let it cook for 11 to 13 minutes or until heated through.
5. Serve immediately garnished with the lemon slices if desired.

NUTRITION

- Calories: 171
- Total Fat: 7.8 g
- Carbs: 4.8 g
- Protein: 20.3 g

CHAPTER 4.
POULTRY

CHICKEN, SPINACH AND ASPARAGUS SOUP

Preparation Time: 10 minutes
Cooking Time: 30 minutes
Servings: 2

INGREDIENTS

- 2 chicken breasts, cooked, skinless, boneless and shredded
- 1 tablespoon of olive oil
- A pinch of salt and black pepper
- 1 yellow onion, finely chopped
- 2 carrots, chopped
- 3 garlic cloves, minced
- 4 cups of spinach
- 12 asparagus spears, chopped
- 6 cups of low-sodium veggie stock
- Zest of ½ lime, grated
- 1 handful cilantro, chopped

DIRECTIONS

1. Heat a pot with the oil over medium heat, add onions, stir and cook for 5 minutes.
2. Add the carrots, garlic and asparagus, stir and cook for 5 minutes.
3. Add the spinach, salt, pepper, stock, and chicken, stir and cook for 20 minutes.
4. Add the lime zest and cilantro. Stir soup again, ladle into bowls and serve.
5. Enjoy!

NUTRITION
- Calories: 245
- Fat: 2 g
- Fiber: 3 g
- Carbs: 5 g
- Protein: 6 g

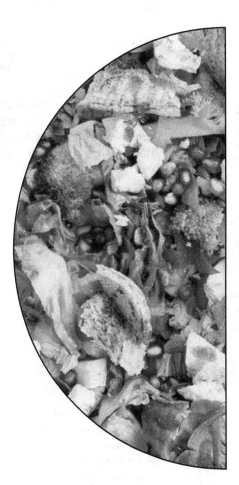

CHICKEN AND BROCCOLI SALAD

Preparation Time: 10 minutes
Cooking Time: 10 minutes
Servings: 2

INGREDIENTS

- 3 medium chicken breasts, skinless, boneless, and cut into thin strips
- 12 ounces of broccoli florets, roughly chopped
- 5 tablespoon of olive oil
- A pinch of salt and black pepper
- 2 tablespoon of vinegar
- 1 and ½ cups of peaches, pitted and sliced
- 1 tablespoon of chives, chopped
- 2 bacon slices, cooked and crumbled

DIRECTIONS

1. In a salad bowl, mix 4 tablespoon of oil with vinegar, salt, pepper, broccoli, peaches, and toss.
2. Heat a pan with the rest of the oil over medium-high heat, add chicken, season with salt and pepper, cook for 5 minutes on each side, transfer to the salad bowl, add bacon and chives, toss and serve.
3. Enjoy!

NUTRITION
- Calories: 210
- Fat: 12 g
- Fiber: 3 g
- Carbs: 10 g
- Protein: 23 g

GARLICKY ZUCCHINI-TURKEY CASSEROLE

Preparation Time: 10 minutes
Cooking Time: 40 minutes
Servings: 2

INGREDIENTS

- 1 tablespoon of oil
- 1 white onion, chopped
- 2 cloves of garlic, minced
- 1-pound cooked turkey meat, shredded
- A dash of rosemary
- 1 zucchini, chopped
- 1 carrot, peeled and chopped
- ½ cup water
- Pepper to taste

DIRECTIONS

1. Preheat oven to 400 ºF.
2. Grease an oven-safe casserole dish with oil.
3. Mix the onion, garlic, turkey, pepper, salt, and rosemary in a bowl.
4. Pour into prepared casserole dish.
5. Sprinkle carrot on top, followed by zucchini, and then pour water over the mixture.
6. Cover the dish with a foil and bake for 25 minutes or until bubbly hot.
7. Remove foil, return to oven, and broil the top for 2 minutes on high.
8. Let it rest for 10 minutes.
9. Serve and enjoy.

NUTRITION

- Calories: 250
- Carbs: 5.7 g
- Protein: 32.9 g
- Fat: 10.0 g
- Saturated Fat: 2.8 g
- Sodium: 88 mg

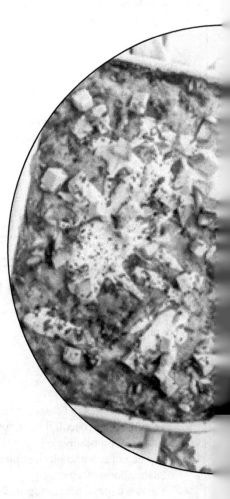

CASSEROLE A LA CHICKEN ENCHILADA

Preparation Time: 10 minutes
Cooking Time: 6 hours
Servings: 2

INGREDIENTS

- 5 pitted dates
- 3 tablespoons of olive oil
- ¼ cup of chili powder
- 1 cup of water
- 1 cup of tomato paste
- 1 teaspoon of ground cumin
- 1 teaspoon of dried oregano
- Salt and pepper to taste
- 2 pounds of chicken breasts, cut into strips
- 1 sweet potato, scrubbed and chopped

DIRECTIONS

1. In a blender or food processor, place the dates, olive oil, chili powder, water, tomato paste, cumin, and oregano. Season with salt and pepper to taste. Pulse until smooth. This will be the enchilada sauce.
2. On the Crock-Pot, place the chicken breasts and sweet potatoes on the bottom of the pot.
3. Pour over chicken the enchilada sauce.
4. Close the lid, press the low settings, and adjust the cooking time to 6 hours.
5. Serve and enjoy.

NUTRITION

- Calories: 240
- Carbs: 12.2 g
- Protein: 30.2 g
- Fat: 8.0 g
- Saturated Fat: 2.7 g
- Sodium: 204 mg

CILANTRO-COCONUT CHICKEN STEW

Preparation Time: 10 minutes
Cooking Time: 30 minutes
Servings: 2

INGREDIENTS

- 1 whole chicken, around 2-lbs
- 1 can of light coconut milk
- 1 cup of water
- ½ fresh cilantro, chopped
- 1 tablespoon of ginger
- 1 teaspoon of cumin
- 1 teaspoon of coriander
- ½ teaspoon of salt
- ½ teaspoon of curry
- 1 lemon, juice extracted

DIRECTIONS

1. Place a heavy bottomed pot on a medium-high fire.
2. Add all the ingredients except for coconut milk. Mix well.
3. Bring to a boil. Once boiling, lower the fire to a simmer and cook for 20 minutes.
4. Stir in coconut milk. Continue simmering for another 10 minutes.
5. Serve and enjoy.

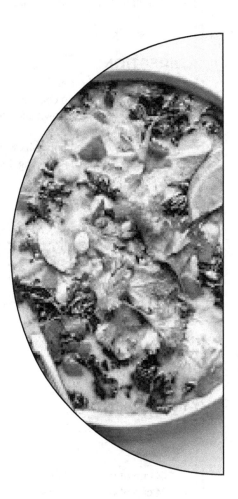

TURKEY LEGS IN THAI SAUCE

Preparation Time: 10 minutes
Cooking Time: 30 minutes
Servings: 2

INGREDIENTS

- 1 ½ pound of large turkey legs
- 1 can of light coconut milk
- 1 cup of water
- 1 ½ teaspoon of lemon juice
- ¼ cup of cilantro, chopped
- Pepper to taste

DIRECTIONS

1. Place a heavy bottomed pot on a medium-high fire.
2. Add all the ingredients except for coconut milk. Mix well.
3. Bring to a boil. Once boiling, lower the fire to a simmer and cook for 20 minutes.
4. Stir in the coconut milk. Continue simmering for another 10 minutes.
5. Serve and enjoy.

FILLING TURKEY CHILI RECIPE

Preparation Time: 10 minutes
Cooking Time: 25 minutes
Servings: 2

INGREDIENTS

- 1 tablespoon of olive oil
- 1-pound of ground turkey
- 1 onion, chopped
- 1 green bell pepper, seeded and chopped
- 3 carrots, peeled and chopped
- 2 stalks of celery, sliced thinly
- 1 cup of chopped tomatoes
- 3 Poblano chilies, chopped
- ½ cup of water
- 3 tablespoons of chili powder
- 1 ½ teaspoon of ground cumin
- Pepper to taste

DIRECTIONS

1. Place a heavy bottomed pot on medium-high fire and heat for 3 minutes.
2. Add the oil; swirl to coat bottom and sides of the pot, and heat for a minute.
3. Stir in the turkey. Brown and crumble for 8 minutes. Season generously with pepper. Discard excess fat.
4. Add all the ingredients. Mix well.
5. Bring to a boil. Once boiling, lower the fire to a simmer and cook for 10 minutes.
6. Serve and enjoy.

NUTRITION

- Calories: 175
- Carbs: 8.7 g
- Protein: 16.4 g
- Fat: 9.1 g
- Saturated Fat: 2.0 g
- Sodium: 188 mg

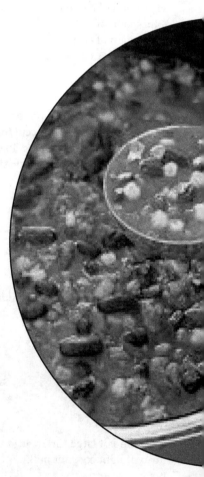

CHICKEN MEATLOAF WITH A TROPICAL TWIST

Preparation Time: 10 minutes
Cooking Time: 45 minutes
Servings: 2

INGREDIENTS

- 1/8 teaspoon of salt
- 1/8 teaspoon of pepper
- 2 eggs
- ¼ cup of parsley, chopped
- ¼ cup of coconut flakes
- ½ tablespoons of jalapeno, seeded and diced
- ½ cups of diced mango
- 1 cup of yellow bell pepper, diced
- 1-pound of ground chicken
- 1 tablespoon of oil

DIRECTIONS

1. Preheat oven to 400 °F and lightly grease a loaf pan with oil.
2. In a large bowl, mix the remaining ingredients.
3. Evenly spread in a prepared pan and cover the pan with foil.
4. Pop in the oven and bake for 30 minutes.
5. Remove foil and broil the top for 3 minutes.
6. Let it sit for 10 minutes.
7. Serve and enjoy.

NUTRITION

- Calories: 301
- Carbs: 8 g
- Protein: 25 g
- Fat: 19 g
- Saturated Fat: 4.6 g
- Sodium: 215 mg

CHAPTER 5.
MEAT

PORK AND LIME SCALLIONS

Preparation Time: 10 minutes
Cooking Time: 30 minutes
Servings: 2

INGREDIENTS

- 2 tablespoons of lime juice
- 4 scallions, chopped
- 1 pound of pork stew meat, cubed
- 2 garlic cloves, minced
- 2 tablespoons of olive oil
- Black pepper to the taste
- ½ cup of low-sodium veggie stock
- 1 tablespoon of cilantro, chopped

DIRECTIONS

1. Heat a pan with the oil over medium heat, add the scallions and the garlic, toss and cook for 5 minutes.
2. Add the meat, toss and cook for 5 minutes more.
3. Add the rest of the ingredients, bring to a simmer and cook over medium heat for 20 minutes.
4. Divide the mix between plates and serve.

NUTRITION

- Calories: 273
- Fat: 22.4 g
- Fiber: 5 g
- Carbs: 12.5 g
- Protein: 18 g

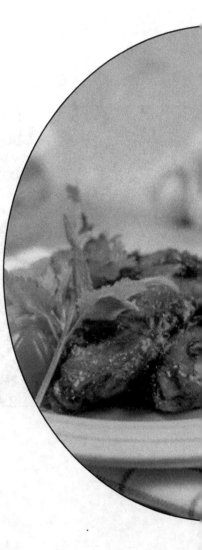

BALSAMIC PORK

Preparation Time: 10 minutes
Cooking Time: 30 minutes
Servings: 2

INGREDIENTS

- 1 red onion, sliced
- 1 pound of pork stew meat, cubed
- 2 red chilies, chopped
- 2 tablespoons of balsamic vinegar
- ½ cup of coriander leaves, chopped
- Black pepper to the taste
- 2 tablespoons of olive oil
- 1 tablespoon of low-sodium tomato sauce

DIRECTIONS

1. Heat a pan with the oil over medium heat, add the onion and the chilies, toss and cook for 5 minutes.
2. Add the meat, toss and cook for 5 minutes more.
3. Add the rest of the ingredients, toss, bring to a simmer and cook over medium heat for 20 minutes more.
4. Divide everything between plates and serve right away.

NUTRITION

- Calories: 331
- Fat: 13.3 g
- Fiber: 5 g
- Carbs: 22.7 g
- Protein: 17 g

PESTO PORK

Preparation Time: 10 minutes
Cooking Time: 36 minutes
Servings: 2

INGREDIENTS

- 2 tablespoons of olive oil
- 2 spring onions, chopped
- 1 pound of pork chops
- 2 tablespoons of basil pesto
- 1 cup of cherry tomatoes, cubed
- 2 tablespoons of low-sodium tomato paste
- ½ cup of parsley, chopped
- ½ cup of low-sodium veggie stock
- Black pepper to the taste

DIRECTIONS

1. Heat a pan with the olive oil over medium-high heat, add the spring onions and the pork chops, and brown for 3 minutes on each side.
2. Add the pesto and the other ingredients, toss gently, bring to a simmer and cook over medium heat for 30 minutes more.
3. Divide everything between plates and serve.

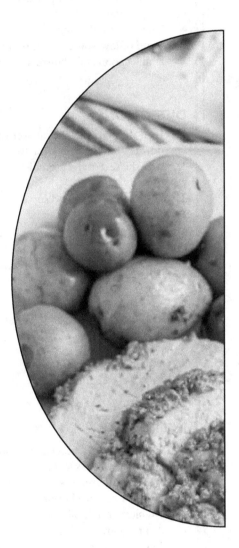

PORK AND PARSLEY PEPPERS

Preparation Time: 10 minutes
Cooking Time: 1 hour
Servings: 2

INGREDIENTS

- 1 green bell pepper, chopped
- 1 red bell pepper, chopped
- 1 yellow bell pepper, chopped
- 1 red onion, chopped
- 1 pound of pork chops
- 1 tablespoon of olive oil
- Black pepper to the taste
- 26 ounces of canned tomatoes, no-salt-added and chopped
- 2 tablespoons of parsley, chopped

DIRECTIONS

1. Grease a roasting pan with the oil, arrange the pork chops inside and add the other ingredients on top.
2. Bake at 390 ºF for 1 hour, divide everything between plates and serve.

CUMIN LAMB MIX

Preparation Time: 10 minutes
Cooking Time: 25 minutes
Servings: 2

INGREDIENTS

- 1 tablespoon of olive oil
- 1 red onion, chopped
- 1 cup of cherry tomatoes, halved
- 1 pound of lamb stew meat, ground
- 1 tablespoon of chili powder
- Black pepper to the taste
- 2 teaspoons of cumin, ground
- 1 cup of low-sodium veggie stock
- 2 tablespoons of cilantro, chopped

DIRECTIONS

1. Heat the pan with the oil over medium-high heat, add the onion, lamb and chili powder, toss and cook for 10 minutes.
2. Add the rest of the ingredients, toss, and cook over medium heat for 15 minutes more.
3. Divide into bowls and serve.

NUTRITION

- Calories: 320
- Fat: 12.7 g
- Fiber: 6 g
- Carbs: 14.3 g
- Protein: 22 g

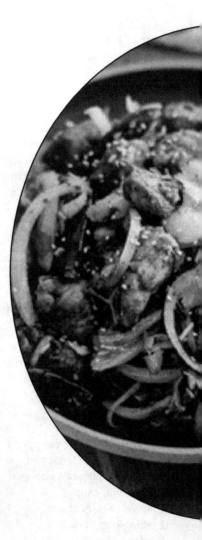

PORK WITH RADISHES AND GREEN BEANS

Preparation Time: 10 minutes
Cooking Time: 35 minutes
Servings: 2

INGREDIENTS

- 1 pound of pork stew meat, cubed
- 1 cup of radishes, cubed
- ½ pound of green beans, trimmed and halved
- 1 yellow onion, chopped
- 1 tablespoon of olive oil
- 2 garlic cloves, minced
- 1 cup of canned tomatoes, no-salt-added and chopped
- 2 teaspoons of oregano, dried
- Black pepper to the taste

DIRECTIONS

1. Heat a pan with the oil over medium-high heat, add the onion and the garlic, toss and cook for 5 minutes.
2. Add the meat, toss and cook for 5 minutes more.
3. Add the rest of the ingredients, bring to a simmer and cook over medium heat for 25 minutes.
4. Divide everything into bowls and serve.

NUTRITION

- Calories: 289
- Fat: 12 g
- Fiber: 8 g
- Carbs: 13.2 g
- Protein: 20 g

FENNEL LAMB AND MUSHROOMS

Preparation Time: 10 minutes
Cooking Time: 40 minutes
Servings: 2

INGREDIENTS

- 1 pound of lamb shoulder, boneless and cubed
- 8 white mushrooms, halved
- 2 tablespoons of olive oil
- 1 yellow onion, chopped
- 2 garlic cloves, minced
- 1 an ½ tablespoons of fennel powder
- Black pepper to the taste
- A bunch of scallions, chopped
- 1 cup of low-sodium veggie stock

DIRECTIONS

1. Heat a pan with the oil over medium heat, add the onion and the garlic, toss and cook for 5 minutes.
2. Add the meat and the mushrooms, toss and cook for 5 minutes more.
3. Add the other ingredients, toss, bring to a simmer and cook over medium heat for 30 minutes.
4. Divide the mix into bowls and serve.

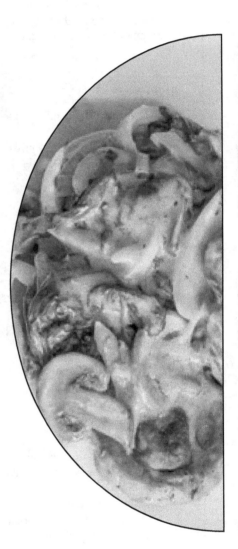

PORK AND SPINACH PAN

Preparation Time: 10 minutes
Cooking Time: 30 minutes
Servings: 2

INGREDIENTS

- 1 pound of pork, ground
- 2 tablespoons of olive oil
- 1 red onion, chopped
- ½ pound of baby spinach
- 4 garlic cloves, minced
- ½ cup of low-sodium veggie stock
- ½ cup of canned tomatoes, no-salt-added, chopped
- Black pepper to the taste
- 1 tablespoon of chives, chopped

DIRECTIONS

1. Heat a pan with the oil over medium-high heat, add the onion and the garlic, toss and cook for 5 minutes.
2. Add the meat, toss and brown for 5 minutes more.
3. Add the rest of the ingredients except the spinach, toss, bring to a simmer, reduce heat to medium and cook for 15 minutes.
4. Add the spinach, toss, cook the mix for another 5 minutes, divide everything into bowls and serve.

PORK WITH AVOCADOS

Preparation Time: 10 minutes
Cooking Time: 15 minutes
Servings: 2

INGREDIENTS

- 2 cups of baby spinach
- 1 pound of pork steak, cut into strips
- 1 tablespoon of olive oil
- 1 cup of cherry tomatoes, halved
- 2 avocados, peeled, pitted and cut into wedges
- 1 tablespoon of balsamic vinegar
- ½ cup of low-sodium veggie stock

DIRECTIONS

1. Heat a pan with the oil over medium-high heat, add the meat, toss and cook for 10 minutes.
2. Add the spinach and the other ingredients, toss, cook for 5 minutes more, divide into bowls and serve.

NUTRITION

- Calories: 390
- Fat: 12.5 g
- Fiber: 4 g
- Carbs: 16.8 g
- Protein: 13.5 g

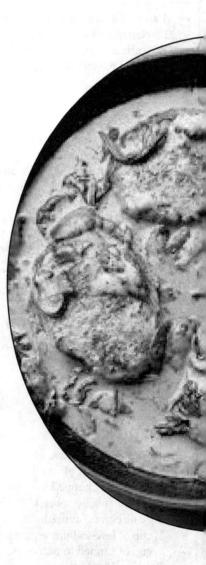

PORK AND SPINACH PAN

Preparation Time: 10 minutes
Cooking Time: 40 minutes
Servings: 2

INGREDIENTS

- 2 pounds of pork stew meat, cut into strips
- 2 green apples, cored and cut into wedges
- 2 garlic cloves, minced
- 2 shallots, chopped
- 1 tablespoon of sweet paprika
- ½ teaspoon of chili powder
- 2 tablespoons of avocado oil
- 1 cup of low-sodium chicken stock
- Black pepper to the taste
- A pinch of red chili pepper flakes

DIRECTIONS

1. Heat a pan with the oil over medium heat; add the shallots and the garlic, toss and sauté for 5 minutes.
2. Add the meat and brown for another 5 minutes.
3. Add the apples and the other ingredients; toss, bring to a simmer and cook over medium heat for 30 minutes more.
4. Divide everything between plates and serve.

NUTRITION

- Calories: 365
- Fat: 7 g
- Fiber: 6 g
- Carbs: 15.6 g
- Protein: 32.4 g

CHAPTER 6.

SALADS & SOUPS

CHESTNUT SOUP

Preparation Time: 10 minutes
Cooking Time: 40 minutes
Servings: 2

INGREDIENTS

- 30 oz. of whole roasted chestnuts
- 1 chopped shallot
- ½ c. of heavy cream
- ½ c. of chicken stock
- 1 chopped leek
- ¼ cup of chopped carrots
- 2 tablespoon of butter
- 1 sprig thyme
- 1 bay leaf
- 1 chopped celery stalk
- ½ teaspoon of nutmeg
- Salt
- Pepper

DIRECTIONS

1. Add the butter, carrot, leek, shallot, and celery in a saucepan over medium heat. Cook for 6-7 minutes or until the vegetables are tender.
2. Add the stock, thyme, bay leaf, chestnuts and bring to boil. Reduce heat and simmer for 25 minutes.
3. Remove from the heat and discard the thyme and bay leaf.
4. Allow to cool slightly and puree using an immersion blender.
5. Heat the soup again as you stir in the cream, nutmeg and season to taste.
6. Cook for 5 minutes more.
7. Serve while still hot.

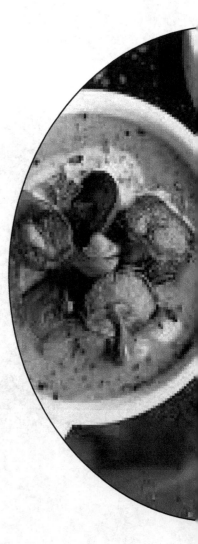

PEPPER POT SOUP

Preparation Time: 10 minutes
Cooking Time: 5 minutes
Servings: 2

INGREDIENTS

- 4 quarts of chicken stock
- 2 diced potatoes
- ½ diced breadfruit
- 1 lb. of diced yam
- ½ lb. of diced cocoa
- 2 crushed garlic cloves
- 2 sprigs of thyme
- 3 chopped green onion
- ½ c. of Coconut Milk
- 10 pimento berries
- 2 chopped callaloo

DIRECTIONS

1. In a reasonable size soup pot, boil 4 quarts of stock.
2. Add garlic, potato, breadfruit, yam, cocoa, and stir.
3. Bring soup to a boil; add thyme, green onion, pimento, callaloo, coconut milk, and pepper.
4. Stir, and cook until done.

QUINOA & AVOCADO SALAD

Preparation Time: 10 minutes
Cooking Time: 5 minutes
Servings: 2

INGREDIENTS

- 1½ c. of cooked quinoa
- 4 oz. of julienned cucumber
- 4 oz. of julienned carrots
- ½ diced avocado
- ½ c. of Brussels sprouts

DIRECTIONS

1. Split your Quinoa into 2 medium bowls.
2. Mix.
3. Top with your cucumber, avocado, and carrot.
4. Add the blanched Brussel Sprouts.
5. Serve and enjoy!

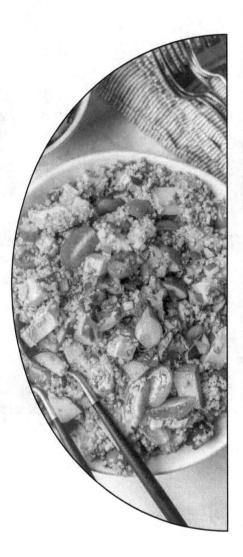

KALE SALAD WITH MIXED VEGETABLES

Preparation Time: 10 minutes
Cooking Time: 5 minutes
Servings: 2

INGREDIENTS
- 1 bunch of chopped Premier kale
- 1 c. of fresh peas
- 2 chopped carrots
- 1 c. of boiled potatoes
- 1 c. of sliced cabbage
- 2 tablespoons of apple cider vinegar
- 1 teaspoon of chili powder
- ½ teaspoon of salt
- 2 tablespoons of coconut oil
- 1 teaspoon of coconut powder

DIRECTIONS
1. Combine all vegetables with kale.
2. Drizzle with vinegar and coconut oil.
3. Season with salt and chili powder.
4. Sprinkle with coconut powder and toss to combine.
5. Add to a serving dish and serve. Enjoy.

CHAPTER 7.
DRESSINGS, SAUCES & SEASONING

ALMOND BUTTER

Preparation Time: 15 minutes
Cooking Time: 15 minutes
Servings: 2

INGREDIENTS

- 2¼ cups of raw almonds
- 1 tablespoon of coconut oil
- ¾ teaspoon of salt
- 4-6 drops of liquid stevia
- ½ teaspoon of ground cinnamon

DIRECTIONS

1. Preheat the oven to 325 ºF.
2. Arrange the almonds onto a rimmed baking sheet in an even layer.
3. Bake for about 12-15 minutes.
4. Remove the almonds from the oven and let them cool completely.
5. In a food processor fitted with a metal blade, place the almonds and pulse until a fine meal forms.
6. Add the coconut oil, salt, and pulse for about 6-9 minutes.
7. Add the stevia, cinnamon, and pulse for about 1-2 minutes.
8. You can preserve this almond butter in the refrigerator by placing it into an airtight container.

NUTRITION

- Calories: 226
- Net Carbs: 3.2 g
- Carbohydrates: 7.8 g
- Fiber: 4.6 g
- Protein: 7.6 g
- Fat: 20.1 g
- Sugar: 1.5 g
- Sodium: 291 mg

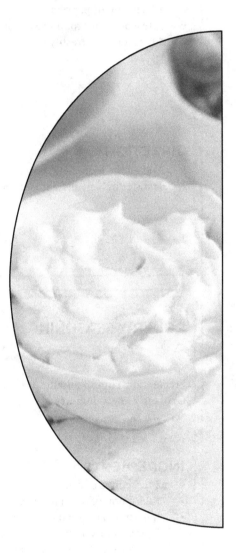

MAYONNAISE

Preparation Time: 10 minutes
Cooking Time: 0 minutes
Servings: 2

INGREDIENTS

- 2 organic egg yolks
- 3 teaspoons of fresh lemon juice, divided
- 1 teaspoon of mustard
- ½ cup of coconut oil, melted
- ½ cup of olive oil
- Salt and ground black pepper, as required -optional

DIRECTIONS

1. Place the egg yolks, 1 teaspoon of lemon juice, and mustard in a blender and pulse until combined.
2. While the motor is running gradually, add both oils and pulse until a thick mixture forms.
3. Add the remaining lemon juice, salt, and black pepper and pulse until well combined.
4. You can preserve this mayonnaise in the refrigerator by placing into an airtight container.
5. Note: if the mayonnaise seems too thin, slowly add more oils while the motor is running until thick.

NUTRITION

- Calories: 193
- Net Carbs: 0.2 g
- Carbohydrates: 0.3 g
- Fiber: 0.1 g
- Protein: 0.6 g
- Fat: 22 g
- Sugar: 0.1 g
- Sodium: 17 mg

SEASONED SALT

Preparation Time: 5 minutes
Cooking Time: 0 minutes
Servings: 28

INGREDIENTS

- ¼ cup of kosher salt
- ½ teaspoon of onion powder
- 1 teaspoon of garlic powder
- 1 teaspoon of paprika
- ½ teaspoon of ground red pepper
- 4 teaspoons of freshly ground black pepper

DIRECTIONS

1. Add all the ingredients to a bowl and stir to combine.
2. Transfer into an airtight jar to preserve.

NUTRITION

- Calories: 2
- Net Carbs: 0.4 g
- Carbohydrates: 0.6 g
- Fiber: 0.2 g
- Protein: 0.1 g
- Fat: 0.1 g
- Sugar: 0.1 g
- Sodium: 1500 mg

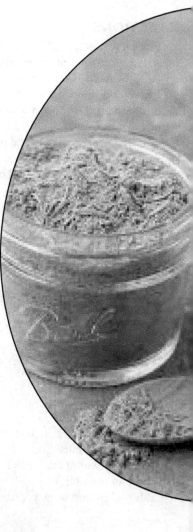

POULTRY SEASONING

Preparation Time: 5 minutes
Cooking Time: 0 minutes
Servings: 2

INGREDIENTS

- 2 teaspoons of dried sage, crushed finely
- 1 teaspoon of dried marjoram, crushed finely
- ¾ teaspoon of dried rosemary, crushed finely
- 1½ teaspoons of dried thyme, crushed finely
- ½ teaspoon of ground nutmeg
- ½ teaspoon of ground black pepper

DIRECTIONS

1. 1. Add all the ingredients to a bowl and stir to combine.
2. 2. Transfer into an airtight jar to preserve.

NUTRITION

- Calories: 2
- Net Carbs: 0.2 g
- Carbohydrates: 0.4 g
- Fiber: 0.2 g
- Protein: 0.1 g
- Fat: 0.1 g
- Sugar: 0 g
- Sodium: 0 mg

CHAPTER 8.

SNACKS

EGG CHIPS

Preparation Time: 15 minutes
Cooking Time: 15 minutes
Servings: 2

INGREDIENTS

- 4 eggs whites
- 2 tablespoons of parmesan, shredded
- 1/2 tablespoon of water
- Salt and black pepper to the taste

DIRECTIONS

1. In a bowl, mix the egg whites with salt, pepper, and water and whisk well.
2. Spoon this into a muffin pan, sprinkle cheese on top, introduce in the oven at 400 °F and bake for 15 minutes.
3. Transfer the egg white chips to a platter and serve with a dip on the side.

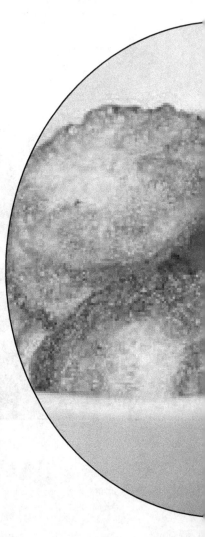

NUTRITION

- Calories: 120
- Fat: 2 g
- Fiber: 1 g
- Carbs: 2 g
- Protein: 7 g

CHEESE BURGER MUFFINS

Preparation Time: 40 minutes
Cooking Time: 20 minutes
Servings: 2

INGREDIENTS

- 1/2 cup of flaxseed meal
- 1 teaspoon of baking powder
- 1/4 cups of sour cream
- 1/2 cup of almond flour
- 2 eggs
- Salt and black pepper to the taste

For the filling:
- 1/2 teaspoon of onion powder
- 2 tablespoons of tomato paste
- 1/2 teaspoon of garlic powder
- 1/2 cup of cheddar cheese, grated
- 16 ounces of beef, ground
- 2 tablespoons of mustard
- Salt and black pepper to the taste

DIRECTIONS

1. In a bowl, mix almond flour with a flaxseed meal, salt, pepper, baking powder, and whisk.
2. Add the eggs and sour cream and stir very well.
3. Divide this into a greased muffin pan and press well using your fingers.
4. Heat a pan over medium-high heat; add beef; stir and brown for a few minutes.
5. Add salt, pepper, onion powder, garlic powder, and tomato paste and stir well.
6. Cook for 5 minutes more and take off the heat.
7. Fill the cupcakes crusts with this mix, introduce in the oven at 350 °F and bake for 15 minutes.
8. Spread cheese on top, introduce in the oven again and bake muffins for 5 minutes more.
9. Serve with mustard and your favorite toppings on top.

NUTRITION

- Calories: 245
- Fat: 16 g
- Fiber: 6 g
- Carbs: 2 g
- Protein: 14 g

CHAPTER 9.

DESSERTS

EASY MACAROONS

Preparation Time: 20 minutes
Cooking Time: 10 minutes
Servings: 2

INGREDIENTS

- 2 cup of coconut; shredded
- 1 teaspoon of vanilla extract
- 4 egg whites
- 2 tablespoons of stevia

DIRECTIONS

1. In a bowl, mix egg whites with stevia and beat using your mixer.
2. Add coconut and vanilla extract and stir.
3. Roll this mixture into small balls and place them on a lined baking sheet.
4. Introduce in the oven at 350 º F and bake for 10 minutes
5. Serve your macaroons cold.

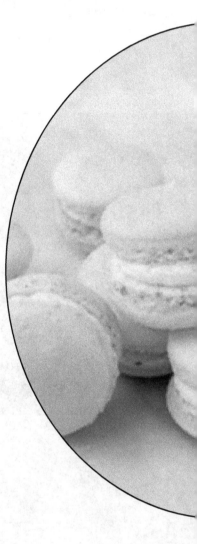

DELICIOUS CHOCOLATE TRUFFLES

Preparation Time: 16 minutes
Cooking Time: 10 minutes
Servings: 2

INGREDIENTS

- 1 cup of sugar-free chocolate chips
- 2 tablespoons of butter
- 2 teaspoons of brandy
- 2 tablespoons of Swerve
- 2/3 cup of heavy cream
- 1/4 teaspoon of vanilla extract
- Cocoa powder

DIRECTIONS

1. Put the heavy cream in a heatproof bowl, add swerve, butter, and chocolate chips; stir, introduce in your microwave and heat up for 1 minute.
2. Leave it aside for 5 minutes; stir well and mix with brandy and vanilla.
3. Stir again, leave aside in the fridge for a couple of hours.
4. Use a melon baller to shape your truffles, roll them in cocoa powder and serve them.

COCONUT PUDDING

Preparation Time: 20 minutes
Cooking Time: 10 minutes
Servings: 2

INGREDIENTS

- 1 2/3 cups of coconut milk
- 1/2 teaspoon of vanilla extract
- 3 egg yolks
- 1 tablespoon of gelatin
- 6 tablespoons of Swerve

DIRECTIONS

1. In a bowl, mix gelatin with 1-tablespoon of coconut milk; stir well and leave aside for now.
2. Put the rest of the milk into a pan and heat up over medium heat.
3. Add the Swerve; stir, and cook for 5 minutes.
4. In a bowl, mix egg yolks with the hot coconut milk and vanilla extract; stir well and return everything to the pan.
5. Cook for 4 minutes, add gelatin and stir well.
6. Divide this into 4 ramekins and keep your pudding in the fridge until you serve it.

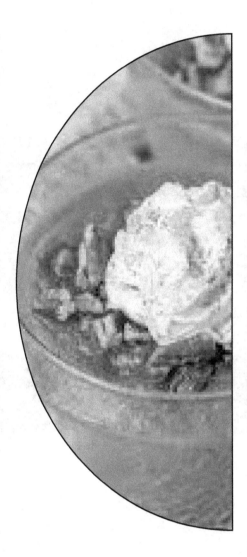

PUMPKIN CUSTARD

Preparation Time: 15 minutes
Cooking Time: 10 minutes
Servings: 2

INGREDIENTS

- 14 ounces of canned coconut milk
- 14 ounces of canned pumpkin puree
- 2 teaspoons of vanilla extract
- 8 scoops of stevia
- 3 tablespoons of Erythritol
- 1 tablespoon of gelatin
- 1/4 cup of warm water
- A pinch of salt
- 1 teaspoon of cinnamon powder
- 1 teaspoon of pumpkin pie spice

DIRECTIONS

1. In a pot, mix pumpkin puree with coconut milk, a pinch of salt, vanilla extract, cinnamon powder, stevia, Erythritol, and pumpkin pie spice; stir well and heat up for a couple of minutes
2. In a bowl, mix gelatin and water and stir.
3. Combine the 2 mixtures; stir well, divide custard into ramekins and leave aside to cool down.
4. Keep in the fridge until you serve it.

CHAPTER 10.

EXTRA RECIPES

SHAKSHUKA

Preparation Time: 25 minutes
Cooking Time: 15 minutes
Servings: 2

INGREDIENTS

- 1 chili pepper, chopped
- 1 cup of marinara sauce
- 4 eggs
- Salt and black pepper, to taste
- 1 oz. of feta cheese

DIRECTIONS

1. Preheat the oven to 390 °F.
2. Heat a small ovenproof skillet on medium heat and add marinara sauce and chili pepper.
3. Cook for about 5 minutes and stir in the eggs.
4. Season with salt and black pepper and top with feta cheese.
5. Transfer into the oven and bake for about 15 minutes.
6. Remove from the oven and serve hot Shakshuka.

NUTRITION

- Calories: 273
- Total Fat: 15.1 g
- Saturated Fat: 5.7 g
- Cholesterol: 342 mg
- Sodium: 794 mg
- Total Carbohydrates: 18.7 g
- Dietary Fiber: 3.3 g
- Total Sugars: 12.4 g
- Protein: 15.4 g

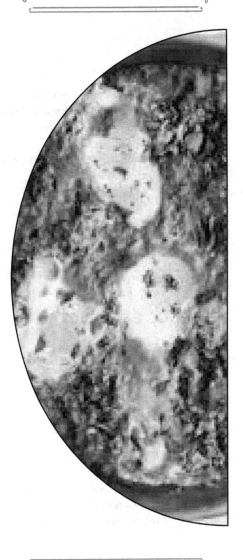

ROOIBOS TEA LATTE

Preparation Time: 20 minutes
Cooking Time: 15 minutes
Servings: 2

INGREDIENTS

- 2 bags of rooibos tea
- 1 cup of water
- 1 tablespoon of grass fed butter
- 1 scoop of collagen peptides
- ¼ cup of full fat canned coconut milk

DIRECTIONS

1. Put the tea bags in boiling water and steep for about 5 minutes.
2. Discard the tea bags and stir in butter and coconut milk.
3. Pour this mixture into a blender and blend until smooth.
4. Add the collagen to the blender and blend at low speed until incorporated.
5. Pour into a mug to serve hot or chilled as desired.

NUTRITION

- Calories: 283
- Total Fat: 23.5 g
- Saturated Fat: 18.3 g
- Cholesterol: 31 mg
- Sodium: 21 mg
- Total Carbohydrates: 3.4 g
- Dietary Fiber: 0 g
- Total Sugars: 2.4 g
- Protein: 15 g

FETA AND PESTO OMELET

Preparation Time: 10 minutes
Cooking Time: 15 minutes
Servings: 2

INGREDIENTS

- 3 eggs
- 2 tablespoons of butter
- 1 oz. of feta cheese
- Salt and black pepper, to taste
- 1 tablespoon of pesto

DIRECTIONS

1. Heat the butter in a pan and allow it to melt.
2. Whisk the eggs in a bowl and pour into the pan.
3. Cook for about 3 minutes until done, and add feta cheese and pesto.
4. Season with salt and black pepper and fold it over.
5. Cook for another 5 minutes until the feta cheese is melted and dish out onto a platter to serve.

NUTRITION

- Calories: 178
- Total Fat: 16.2 g
- Saturated Fat: 8.1 g
- Cholesterol: 194 mg
- Sodium: 253 mg
- Total Carbohydrates: 1.1 g
- Dietary Fiber: 0.1 g
- Total Sugars: 1.1 g
- Protein: 7.5 g

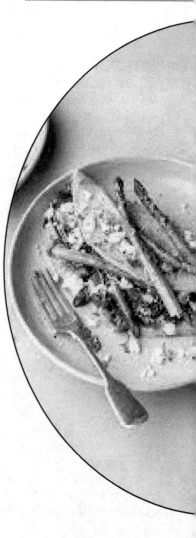

EGGS BENEDICT

Preparation Time: 25 minutes
Cooking Time: 15 minutes
Servings: 2

INGREDIENTS

- 4 Oopsie rolls
- 4 eggs
- 4 Canadian bacon slices, cooked and crisped
- 1 tablespoon of white vinegar
- 1 teaspoon of chives

DIRECTIONS

1. Boil water with vinegar and create a whirlpool in it with a wooden spoon.
2. Break an egg in a cup and place in the boiling water for about 3 minutes.
3. Repeat with the rest of the eggs and dish out onto a platter.
4. Place Oopsie rolls on the plates and top with bacon slices.
5. Put the poached eggs onto bacon slices and garnish with chives to serve.

NUTRITION

- Calories: 190
- Total Fat: 13.5 g
- Saturated Fat: 5.8 g
- Cholesterol: 275 mg
- Sodium: 587 mg
- Total Carbohydrates: 1.5 g
- Dietary Fiber: 0 g
- Total Sugars: 0.6 g
- Protein: 15.3 g

CPSIA information can be obtained
at www.ICGtesting.com
Printed in the USA
LVHW061124300821
696428LV00014B/376